Blessed & Grateful.

Introduction

So, you want to be a runner….but you've never ran before (or it's been a few years/decades) and you have no idea where to start. You're overwhelmed at the thought of even picking out a pair of running shoes.

The thing is, you're not the first person to start from scratch -- everyone has to start somewhere. Think you're too old? Think again, the average age for male marathoners is 40, while the average woman running a marathon is 37 years old [1]. What other excuse do you have? Whatever it is, lock it up and give this thing a try -- you might surprise yourself.

Beginning a running program may seem overwhelmingly complicated, but it's only as complicated as you make it. Whether you're looking to run your first 5K or you have your sights set on a longer race, I'm going to break down the basics of running and serve it up over easy.

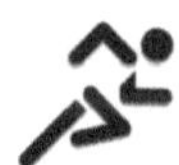

Why Should you Run?

If you're reading this, you're obviously interested in running. But, just in case you're still not completely sold, let me tell you a little bit about why running is so great.

Fitness

Perhaps the most obvious benefit of running is the fact that it will improve your level of fitness. Even if you go at a pace that could be rivaled by a baby sloth, your fitness will improve. Any activity that pushes you beyond your current level of existence will improve your fitness capacity. Maybe right now taking a flight of stairs feels like completing an Ironman -- with a few weeks of running under your belt, it will feel more like a Spartan Sprint and, with continued training, eventually it won't even phase you.

Make Your Heart Happy

What works harder than your air-sucking lungs and Jell-O legs during a run? That would be your heart. As you take stride after stride, your ticker is working overtime to get oxygen-rich blood (courtesy of your lungs) distributed to your working leg muscles. Running on a regular basis will make your heart stronger and more efficient at pumping. As its efficiency increases, your heart rate will actually begin to decrease, which means you'll have a lower heart rate while maintaining a pace that before would've nearly killed you. You'll also develop a lower resting heart rate [2], allowing your heart to actually rest when you're resting.

Fat Loss

Because running, at any speed, results in calorie usage, there is a good chance you'll experience some level of fat loss -- as long as you don't completely undo all that work when you step foot in the kitchen. In fact, one 12-week running program was shown to significantly reduce waist circumference and body fat percentage [2]. It should be noted, while long slow runs have the potential to burn several hundred calories, they're not necessarily your best bet if fat loss is your goal.

High-Intensity Intermittent Training, more commonly referred to as HIIT, is the more productive route to take for fat loss. HIIT involves completing bouts of high-intensity sprints, followed by a recovery period and repeating. It has been shown to significantly lower insulin resistance, enhance skeletal muscle fat oxidation, and improve glucose tolerance [3] -- all three of which are very important for long-term fat loss. HIIT has also proven to be more effective than steady slow exercise at significantly reducing total body fat and subcutaneous fat (the fat under the skin) in the trunk and legs [4]. I'd like to add that as your body becomes more efficient at fueling your runs, you're ultimately going to burn fewer and fewer calories with the same workout. Keep your body guessing by changing up your run distance, pace, terrain, and implementing HIIT workouts, to keep the calorie burn up.

Better Health

While you're getting in better shape, making your heart happy and losing fat, your body is also enduring several more positive changes on the health side. For starters, by beginning a running program that increases your fitness level, you can significantly reduce your risk of premature death -- by 44% according to one study [8]. If that's not enough, running on a regular basis can also help decrease your risk of developing Type 2 diabetes [9], cancer (especially breast and colon) [11], osteoporosis [12] (that constant pounding makes for strong bones), and it also helps with the management of diabetes [10]. Regular aerobic activity also helps to decrease levels of bad cholesterol and triglycerides while simultaneously increasing good cholesterol [13].

Boost Your Energy

As your fitness and endurance improve with your running program, you'll notice your energy levels increasing throughout the day. It's pretty obvious if you think about it -- if you can run a few miles, you should definitely be able to keep up with your kids on the playground. When your body gets more efficient at delivering blood and oxygen during your workout, it also gets better during rest, which means it takes considerably less energy to keep the lights on than it did before you made the decision to begin running.

Decrease Your Desire to Throat Punch

How often do you fantasize about drilling someone right in the windpipe? Depending on your work environment or daily routine, this could be a very common occurrence. Instead of acting on your urge, go for a run. Regular cardio exercise, such as running, has been shown to improve mood, improve sleep (making you less irritable during the day), relieve stress [5], improve self-esteem and cognitive function [6], and reduce anxiety and depression [7]. All-in-all, a daily run can make you a happier, more understanding and a less volatile individual -- a win for everyone!

I think it's safe to say, scheduling in a few runs a week would be very beneficial for your body, your health and your sanity. Your spouse and co-workers can thank me later.

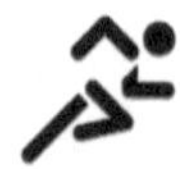

What do Runners Wear?

Hopefully by now, you agree that running is indeed a good idea. Perfect! Now, onto more important things -- like what to wear.

The Mainstays

Runners wear all sorts of different clothing; it really depends on function and preference. Generally speaking, you can go with simple running shorts/leggings and a t-shirt or tank top. Ideally, you'll want a moisture-wicking material to keep you comfortable, but an old cotton t-shirt will work fine (it will just absorb and hold the sweat).

Socks & Compression

A well-made moisture-wicking sock will keep your feet comfortable and blisters to a minimum. For bounce control, ladies, you'll want a good sports bra and guys, compression shorts are a must.

Shoes

As a runner, the most important aspect of your wardrobe to consider is your shoes. A bad shoe choice can turn your dreams of being a runner into a nightmare. The perfect running shoe is not only built for comfort but also to address and accommodate any issues you may have with your foot strike and gate. To be honest, I believe these things should be dealt with by a sports medicine professional before you begin a running program. However, most of the time people just go for it.

So, how do you find the right shoe? First off, don't buy them off the internet (unless you've already tried them on in-store and know you love them). You need to physically try on shoes to make sure they properly accommodate your foot-width and arch, and actually fit your foot. I recommend going to a store with trained specialists who can help you find and fit the perfect shoe for you.

Gear

Now that we've covered the basic necessities, let's get to the stuff that's fun to spend our money on. If you're running any amount of distance, you'll need some sort of hydration source. You can opt for a backpack like a Camelbak, or a hydration belt with small bottles of water strapped in. Both of these options generally give you a little room to store gels or gummies, which we'll touch on later.

Head and eye protection are also important. I suggest always donning a hat or visor with some sweet shades -- you'll look and stay cooler. Winter time runners should definitely not leave the house without a beanie or buff.

If you're heading out for a trail run, a set of tall socks or a pair of gators are a good idea to keep your legs protected from the brush and keep debris from getting inside your shoes.

Some people have issues with "chub rub" as the hubs and I like to call it (we both experience it from time to time). This little darling occurs when your thighs rub together, cause chafing and get sore. This is a common problem and, thankfully, there's a solution. Body Glide is one such solution -- it comes in a stick that looks like deodorant. Just rub it on the problem area(s) and you'll have smooth sailing during your run.

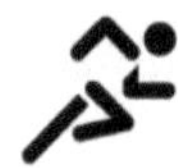

Run the Right Way

While running is a natural movement all humans are capable of, it doesn't always come easy to us. Yes, some people are naturally good and graceful runners, but then there are others who look like baby giraffes taking their first steps. If you fall into the latter category, let's take a few minutes to discuss how to run the right way, with good form and not get hurt.

While you should by no means over-think your form, you definitely want to be aware of your body. We'll start at the top and work our way down.

Keep your head up and look straight ahead toward the horizon, this will keep your airway open and allow you to see what's coming.

Avoid clenching your jaw while you run -- keep it relaxed so you can easily inhale through your mouth.

Your upper body should be relaxed and open. Keep your elbows bent to 90 degrees, your torso upright, hands relaxed and chest big (allowing your chest to collapse forward will reduce your lung capacity, something we definitely do not want).

Keep your arms close to your sides (avoid swinging them from side-to-side) and rotate at the shoulders.

Keep your stride short and quick. Taking steps that are too long for your body (over-striding) is a good way to get hurt.

Land mid-foot. Running on your toes will overwork your calves and lead to fatigue and potential injury, while striking the ground with your heel causes unnecessary shock impact to your body and wastes a lot of energy.

Keep your toes pointed forward, not turned out or in.

Don't bounce when you step. Keep your energy moving in a forward direction to prevent wasting energy going up and down.

Don't Forget to Breathe

Some people will naturally develop an efficient breathing pattern while running. Others will hold their breath, breathe too quickly or breathe too shallowly. Avoid overthinking things. You can't run without oxygen, so just let it in.

Mouth breathing is acceptable and preferred while you run. Use every resource you have -- mouth and nose -- to get air in. Some people breathe in through their nose and exhale through their mouth. I tried that once and almost went down. How they do it? I have no idea. Let's just focus on keeping both airways open.

As you run, focus on belly breathing -- breathing deep into your belly. You will not get enough oxygen if you rely solely on your chest to pull air in. Take nice slow, deep breaths and exhale in a similar fashion. If you're not a natural belly breather, practice while standing or sitting. Place your hand on your belly so you can feel it expanding and contracting.

How fast should you breathe? I've found a nice steady rhythm of inhaling for two strides and exhaling for two strides. If this works for you, go for it. If not, play around with it a bit until you find what feels comfortable.

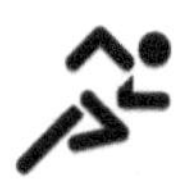

Expectations

I'm not going to sugar coat it for you, when you first start a running program it will suck. If you're not in running shape, it takes work to get there and that interim phase is where you have to dig deep. The good news is, once you begin running, you'll notice each run gets a little easier.

Just remember, you're not going to go out and run a marathon. It's going to take time for your body to adapt, but if you stick with it you CAN run a marathon.

One more great expectation with a new running program -- you will likely experience some muscle soreness, especially in your quads (the front of your legs), hamstrings (back of your legs), and calves. Running uses our leg muscles differently than walking, cycling or using the elliptical, so plan on a at least a little tightness or soreness.

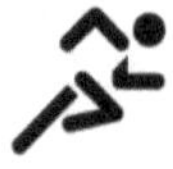

Types of Runs

You may think there's only one type of running, but you'd be wrong. There are actually several types of runs and most of them should eventually make their way into your training regimen. Let's take a look at each type as well as when and why to use them.

Base runs are where you're going to spend most of your training time, especially at the beginning. These runs do exactly what you'd think -- they build a base. These runs develop your running endurance and help strengthen your muscles, tendons and ligaments used repetitively during a run. Base runs are what will build up your body, lungs and heart, and reduce your risk of injuring yourself when you get into the more advanced runs.

For a base run, simply run at your natural pace for the designated amount of time/distance (this will depend on your training program) several times per week.

Long Slow Distance (LSD) runs are your longest of the week and they work to test your endurance. Your LSD run should only occur once per week and when you finish one of these, you should be smoked.

This run doesn't have to be 20 miles, but it does need to be longer than anything you've done all week. So, if you've run two miles, three times this week, your long run could be three to four miles. Definitely take a day off after this run or perform a nice, short, easy recovery run.

Progression runs are just like the name implies -- your pace progresses as you run. These runs are great for beginners to slowly transition to faster paces.

For a three mile run, begin with a nice comfortable pace for the first mile, increase your pace a smidge for the next mile, then finish your last mile with the most intense pace you can maintain.

Fartlek runs (pronounced like it looks) are a great introductory to interval training. How does one fartlek? Simply pick different paces throughout your run to perform for varying distances.

For example, get comfortable in a nice sustainable pace, then pick it up from one street sign to the next; get back to your normal pace for a few minutes, then sprint between the next two street signs. Continue to play around with your pace until your run is completed. That is a fartlek.

Hill repeats are used to build speed, power and strength, and are a great way to introduce higher intensity runs.

Find a nice hill, sprint up it, jog or walk down and repeat. Ideally, it should take 30-45 seconds to get up the hill.

Tempo runs (also known as threshold runs) are performed at just below your lactate threshold -- in other words just below the spot where you feel like you're going to die. These runs are shorter runs, especially for beginners, and are meant to increase your ability to maintain this fast pace while also increasing said pace.

Start with a five to 10-minute tempo run once per week, working your way up to 20 to 30 minutes.

Interval runs are performed by alternating a very fast pace (usually a sprint) with lower intensity or complete rest. These runs are usually performed on a track so that you have a solid, safe surface to sprint on and you can easily measure your distance. Interval runs help increase your running speed, fatigue resistance and pain tolerance (yes, they're that much fun).

Don't worry about intervals until you've been training awhile, at which point you could work them in every couple of weeks. When you do them, begin with shorter distances like 200 to 400-meter sprints followed by 200-meter recovery jog or walk.

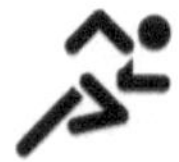

Cross-Training

If you're going to be a runner, it's obviously important that you run, but it's also important that you don't. Running every day is a good way to set yourself up for injury. Yes, there are some athletes who can do it, but they're the exception to the rule and most have been running for years, so they're adapted to the stresses. You should plan on running three to four days per week. Choose one day for recovery and the other days should consist of an activity other than running.

Effective cross-training options include rowing, cycling, swimming, hiking, yoga, Pilates and, my personal favorite, strength training. While I think the other cardio-type activities are great choices, I would recommend making it a point to include yoga and weights into your routine.

Yoga will improve your range of motion and improve flexibility, something runners can always use more of. Plus, keeping your muscles from holding onto chronic tension can help reduce your chance of injury as you progress in your running career.

What about strength training? It may seem like weight lifting and running are on completely different ends of the spectrum and, in a sense, they are. However, if you want to keep your body strong and healthy, you should consider including weights into your training program.

Strength training has been shown to increase the rate of force development (how fast your foot leaves the ground), increase running economy (how efficiently your body produces and uses energy while running), increase maximal speed [14], and increase your time to exhaustion [15]. If you're concerned the weights will turn you into a running hulk, don't worry, you'll be fine. The benefits on running performance that tend to accompany strength training do not include added bulk [16]. As an added bonus, these benefits can be accrued with only two sessions per week [16]! To learn more about strength training, check out my first book Strength Training Over Easy.

During your cross-training workouts, take the time to work your core. A strong core is to a runner what armor is to a knight. Seriously. A weak core could spell disaster for any dreams you may have to be a runner. Core strength and stability cannot only make you a faster runner [17], it can also play an important role in injury prevention [18]. Exercises that target your rectus abdominis (the front of your stomach), your obliques (the sides of your stomach), your lower back, and all three groups of gluteal muscles (think squats, leg lifts to the side, clam exercises, etc.), will help keep your hips, knees and ankles aligned and stable and your risk of injury low.

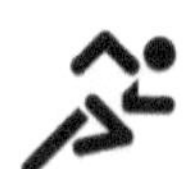

Have a Plan and Track Your Progress

When you start a running program, have a plan. Yes, you can just start running to run, but you might burn out without a goal to focus on. I'm not saying you have to run a race, but putting one in your sites is a surefire way to get you moving every day. In addition to your long-term goals (like said race), make short-term goals such as, "run three times per week," "work up to one mile over the next two weeks," "run on Monday, Wednesday, Friday and Sunday this week first thing in the morning."

Keep your goals specific, measurable, attainable, realistic and timely (SMART) to keep you looking forward to the next challenge.

Each week, make it a point to track your progress. It can sometimes get discouraging, but looking back on where you started and how far you've come goes a long way to boost your self-esteem. Keep track of how far or long you actually run each trip out, or time yourself on a loop you run often. You'll be amazed how much faster/farther you can go after just a few weeks.

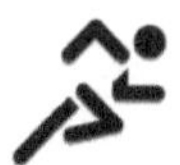

Weather Considerations

Wouldn't it be nice if every run took place on a not too hot, not too cold day? It would be awesome, but unfortunately we only get a handful of "perfect" running days every year. It's not a big deal -- any day can be a running day, as long as you prepare accordingly. Let's take a minute to discuss running in the two extremes -- cold and heat.

Running in the Cold

I always prefer running in the cold over the heat, except for when we have several feet of snow on the ground. Then I'm out. People often perform better in cooler weather for the simple fact their bodies aren't working double time to keep them from having a heat stroke (more about that in a second), so taking advantage of a cold-weather run may not be a bad idea.

When running in the cold, there's one important factor to consider: layering. Learning how to properly layer your clothes will make running in the cold a much more enjoyable experience. Start with a moisture-wicking base such as merino wool to keep the sweat off of your skin. Next, an insulating layer will keep your body heat in and the cold out. Lastly, choose a weather-resistant shell of some sort. Once you start to warm up, shed a layer to prevent overheating. Once you finish your run, layer back up to keep from chilling too much. Keep in mind, this layering system is most important for your upper body, since your lower body is going to be busy moving. A heavier set of running tights will work fine.

Cold weather running is a great excuse for accessorizing. Hats, gloves, warm technical socks and gaiters are a must. You lose a ton of heat through your head and blood flow to the fingers and toes is limited since your body has better use for that warm oxygen-rich blood. So, to prevent frostbite on the ears and appendages, keep them covered. If it's really cold, you may want to consider a neck gaiter or face mask to put over your mouth, which will help warm up the air before it hits your throat and lungs. The right socks will save your feet from freezing and leg gaiters will keep the snow out of your shoes.

Speaking of shoes, they are another important consideration for cold weather running if your terrain consists of snow and/or ice. When you're running on this kind of surface, it's not a bad idea to invest in a set of shoes with a little more substance. Trail running shoes work well -- the extra traction will give you just what you need to keep from slipping. Another option is to keep what you've already got and just throw on a pair of Yak Trax to give you a little more stability in the snow. Lastly, you can opt for "studded" shoes. Seriously, they make them. These are shoes with little studs in the sole that bite into the ice and snow just like a snow tire to get you through even the worst terrain.

When it's cold outside, it's not a bad idea to warm-up and cool-down indoors rather than standing out in the cold. Get your body prepped for action in the warm comfort of your living room and then stretch it out in front of the fire place or any other warm area after your run.

Lastly, consider investing in a headlamp and reflective belt. Why? If you're running in the cold, that likely means it's winter time and you're dealing with short days and a lot of darkness. Keep yourself visible with lights or reflective gear to avoid getting smoked by an unsuspecting motorist.

Running in the Heat

Running in the heat is a miserable endeavor but it goes with the territory considering many races are held during the summer months. Not to worry, with a little foresight you'll do just fine.

We'll start with clothes -- wear as little as possible and make sure it's moisture-wicking. You do not want a soaked cotton t-shirt slapping against you with every stride. If you prefer to keep covered, there's some really great technical gear on the market for hot environments. Don't leave home without a hat and sunglasses, talk about adding salt to a wound.

The most important consideration with running in the heat is actually overheating. This can occur through dehydration, from actually getting too hot, or a combination of the two. Our bodies divert some of the blood that would normally be delivering oxygen to our muscles, to the skin in an effort to cool it before sending it back to the heart and lungs. This is one reason why running in the heat seems so much harder -- you're working with a smaller blood and oxygen supply.

In addition to cooling our blood, our body has one more trick up its sleeve -- sweating. Sweating is the shuttling of fluid to the skin so that it can be evaporated, thereby cooling the body and enabling us to remain at a somewhat stable body temperature. The only problem is, this takes away from the fluid your body needs to move your blood around. This makes proper hydration a huge necessity in the heat. Always pack water with you and if the humidity is high, consider using some form of electrolyte replacement.

If you're drinking plenty of water and still feel like you're too hot, you probably are. It would be a wise decision to stop running, find some shade, drink some water, pour some water over your head and allow your body temperature to cool down. A heat stroke is not something you want to deal with, especially if you're out on a solo run.

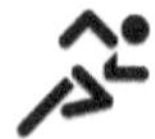

Nutrition

As a beginner, running nutrition isn't a huge deal -- mainly because your runs are going to be on the shorter side. If you opt to pursue longer distances on the other hand, nutrition will become very important.

Food

When is it time to consider fueling? If you're happy running the 5K circuit, you won't need to worry about eating. However, if your runs and races typically exceed the 60-minute mark, you may want to consider downing some calories.

Choosing what kind of calories to eat can be a little tricky, but it's all about trial and error. Find something you like, that doesn't upset your stomach, and go with it. There are a plethora of gels and gummies on the market to choose from, and sports drinks have a few carbohydrates and electrolytes in them to keep you moving for a bit.

Runners eat all sorts of random things, especially the ultra-endurance crowd. To keep it simple, try different foods you have at home -- fruit, pretzels, cereal, jerky or bars. Whatever you go with, try it out several times to make sure your body is good with it -- nothing like having to duck into the brush when a toilet isn't available.

When to eat is just as important as what to eat. A couple of hours prior to your long run, eat something with plenty of carbohydrates and some protein. During your long runs, aim to consume 30-60 grams of carbs every hour. Again, if you're out for a nice 45-minute run, don't worry about eating -- your body can provide its own energy for an hour or more.

After a run exceeding 60 minutes, go ahead and refuel with a snack to restore your glycogen stores (what your muscles use for energy). Again, go with what sounds/feels good -- a PBJ and glass of milk offers a great combo of fat, protein and carbs. If a large snack just does not sound good, find something smaller that you can stomach.

Hydration

While not everyone has to eat during a run, everyone does need water, especially during the hot, humid summer months. Before you even head out the door, make sure you're hydrated -- starting a run in a dehydrated state isn't going to end well for you. Make it a point to swig a couple of cups of water 20 to 30 minutes before you start.

During your run you have two options; 1) trust your body and drink when you're thirsty or 2) hydrate on a schedule. While option one is feasible, it's not always reliable. Sometimes our bodies betray us, cueing the urge to drink only after we're in a state of dehydration. Option two may improve your chances of success by keeping your hydration status at an adequate level.

Do your best to drink four to eight gulps every 15 to 20 minutes during your run. If it's especially hot and/or humid, 10 gulps every 15 minutes may be necessary. Adding a bit of salt to your water can help increase absorption and hydration levels, and make it more palatable.

After your run, there's a very good chance you'll be at some level of dehydration, despite your best efforts. Drink plenty of water or sports drinks once the sweat has dried to ensure you're ready for your next outing, and the rest of the day.

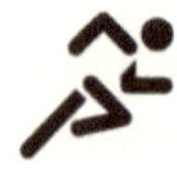

Warm-up and Cool-down

Before you head out the door or crank up the speed on the treadmill, make sure your body is ready to run. This means your muscles need to be warm, your blood vessels need to be dilated, and your heart and lungs need to be ready to work hard. This process takes place during your warm-up, which should always be performed prior to your run.

A warm-up should last five to 10 minutes and consist of light aerobic activity. This could include walking, marching, slow jogging, riding the stationary bike, high knees, butt kicks, skipping, leg swings, lunges and squats. Pick one activity or perform a combination to get your body ready for action.

After your run, give yourself another five to 10 minutes for a nice relaxing cool-down. This period gives your body a chance to transition back to a resting state. Include stretches for your quadriceps, hip flexors, hamstrings, calves and glutes into your cool-down period.

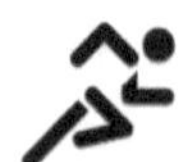

Running Safety and Etiquette

When you go for a run, you're responsible for your personal safety and to make sure you're not obnoxious to others. Here are a few guidelines to keep you as safe and likeable as possible.

Make sure you are fully visible. Wearing camo while running alongside the road would not be a wise decision. If you're running at night, plenty of reflective clothing will make you easier to see. Always ensure someone else knows your running route.

Be aware of your surroundings. Never assume a driver sees you or that a cyclist headed down the path towards you knows you're coming.

Keep your ears open. Yes, music makes running much more enjoyable, but if you can't hear over it, you could miss the sound of a vehicle or another person approaching.

Trust your gut. If a person, environment or situation makes you feel uncomfortable, get out of there!

Carry identification. While it may seem silly to pack an ID on your run, it is a must if something happens. Road ID is a company that makes wearable identification

bracelets, anklets, badges and tags that can display
your name, address, emergency contact and even blood
type -- definitely worth investing in if you're mainly a solo
runner.

Run against traffic. This will give you a chance to get
out of the way if a car happens to veer off the road.

Use the sidewalk. When a sidewalk is available, use it.
This will lessen your chances of getting smoked by a
vehicle, but it may also earn you some dirty looks from
walking pedestrians -- they'll get over it.

Go with the flow. On a running path, run with the flow
of other runners, stay to the right and pass on the left.
Verbally give other runners a heads up when you're
passing -- "on your left" works just fine. On a track, pass
on the right (or the outside lane).

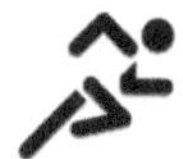

Tips for Getting Started

By now I hope you feel like you have accumulated enough info to take your first spin around the neighborhood. To make your transition into a runner seamless, here are a few tips to keep in mind as you get started.

Start small. Your first trip out doesn't even need to be a mile. Go as far as you can, then walk home. Try and make it a little bit farther next time.

Build gradually. Going too hard too fast will most definitely result in some sort of injury -- or in you flat out hating the idea of running. When ramping up, choose to increase your distance, time OR frequency, not all three. Avoid increasing your mileage by more than 10% each week.

Stick with the basics. Make most of your runs, base runs with one long run per week. Remember, a long run is relative to your current training program -- not to a marathoners training program.

Don't run every day. Give your body time to adapt and recover from your runs. Heading out three to four times per week is plenty.

Stay strong. Use weights to strengthen your muscles and connective tissues -- this will drastically reduce your

risk of injury. A strong and stable core should be a top
priority.

Don't forget to stretch. Keep your muscles supple and
flexible so you can handle what the road throws at you.

Have fun and smile. Life is good. Running is good.
Enjoy yourself.

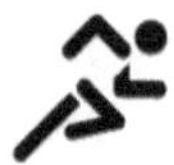

Conclusion

Now that you have the inside scoop on running, I hope you feel like it's something you can take on. Whether you hit the pavement in hopes of completing your first road race or you begin your journey to improve your health, keep in mind it is doable and it is worth it.

Run strong, friends.

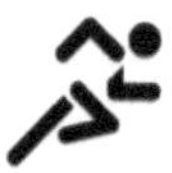

Sample Running Programs

As I mentioned in the book, races make for great goals. If you sign up, you'll HAVE to train or risk not finishing. So, to get you started in your running/racing career, here are a 5K and half-marathon training program. Stick to them and you'll be crossing the finish line strong!

On the days you don't run, choose a cross-training activity of your choice. If you start to get wore down, give yourself one full day of rest per week. And make sure to take a rest day the day before your race.

Sample 8-week 5K Training Program

	Tuesday	Thursday	Sunday
Week 1	Run/walk 1 mile	Run/walk 1 mile	Run/walk 1 mile
Week 2	Run 1 mile	Run 1 mile	Run 1 mile
Week 3	Run/walk 1.5 miles	Run/walk 1.5 miles	Run/walk 1.5 miles
Week 4	Run 1.5 miles	Run 1.5 miles	Run 1.5 miles
Week 5	Run 2 miles	Run 1.5 miles	Run 2 miles
Week 6	Run 2.5 miles	Run 2 miles	Run 2.5 miles
Week 7	Run 3 miles	Run 2.5 miles	Run 3 miles
Week 8	Run 2 miles	Run 1.5 miles	Race Day!

Sample 12-week Half-Marathon Training Program

	Monday	Wednesday	Thursday	Saturday
Week 1	1 mile	1 mile	1 mile	2 miles
Week 2	2 miles	2 miles	2 miles	3 miles
Week 3	2 miles	3 miles	2 miles	4 miles
Week 4	3 miles	2 miles	3 miles	5 miles
Week 5	3 miles	3 miles	3 miles	6 miles
Week 6	4 miles	3 miles	4 miles	7 miles
Week 7	4 miles	4 miles	4 miles	8 miles
Week 8	5 miles	4 miles	5 miles	9 miles
Week 9	5 miles	5 miles	5 miles	10 miles
Week 10	6 miles	5 miles	6 miles	11 miles
Week 11	6 miles	6 miles	6 miles	8 miles
Week 12	2 miles	3 miles	2 miles	Race Day!

References

1) Advanced Solutions International, Inc. "U.S. Road Race Participation Numbers Hold Steady for 2017." U.S. Road Race Participation Numbers Hold Steady for 2017 - 2018 U.S. Running Trends Report. Accessed October 20, 2018. https://runningusa.org/RUSA/News/2018/U.S._Road_Race_Participation_Numbers_Hold_Steady_for_2017.aspx.

2) Kang, Seol-Jung, Eon-Ho Kim, and Kwang-Jun Ko. "Effects of Aerobic Exercise on the Resting Heart Rate, Physical Fitness, and Arterial Stiffness of Female Patients with Metabolic Syndrome." *Journal of Physical Therapy Science* 28, no. 6 (2016): 1764-768. doi:10.1589/jpts.28.1764.

3) Boutcher, Stephen H. "High-Intensity Intermittent Exercise and Fat Loss." *Journal of Obesity* 2011 (2011): 1-10. doi:10.1155/2011/868305.

4) Trapp, E. G., D. J. Chisholm, and S. H. Boutcher. "The Effects of High-intensity Intermittent Exercise Training on Fat Loss and Fasting Insulin Levels of Young Women." *International Journal of Obesity* 32, no. 4 (January 15, 2008): 684-91. doi:10.1038/sj.ijo.0803781.

5) Sharma, A., V. Madaan, and F. Petty. "Exercise for Mental Health." *The Primary Care*

Companion to The Journal of Clinical Psychiatry 8, no. 2 (2006).

6) Callaghan, P. "Exercise: A Neglected Intervention in Mental Health Care?" *Journal of Psychiatric and Mental Health Nursing* 11, no. 4 (2004): 476-83. doi:10.1111/j.1365-2850.2004.00751.x.

7) Guszkowska, M. "The Effects Of Exercise on Anxiety, Depression and Mood." *Phsyciatria Polska* 38, no. 4 (July/August 2004): 611-20.

8) Blair, Steven N. "Changes in Physical Fitness and All-Cause Mortality." *Jama* 273, no. 14 (1995): 1093. doi:10.1001/jama.1995.03520380029031.

9) Helmrich, Susan P., David R. Ragland, Rita W. Leung, and Ralph S. Paffenbarger. "Physical Activity and Reduced Occurrence of Non-Insulin-Dependent Diabetes Mellitus." *New England Journal of Medicine* 325, no. 3 (1991): 147-52. doi:10.1056/nejm199107183250302.

10) Gregg, Edward W., Robert B. Gerzoff, Carl J. Caspersen, David F. Williamson, and K. M. Venkat Narayan. "Relationship of Walking to Mortality Among US Adults With Diabetes." *Archives of Internal Medicine* 163, no. 12 (2003): 1440. doi:10.1001/archinte.163.12.1440.

11) Lee, I. M. "Physical Activity and Cancer Prevention--data from Epidemiologic Studies." *Medicine & Science in Sports & Exercise* 35, no. 11 (November 2003): 1823-827.

12) Warburton, Darren E.r., Norman Gledhill, and Arthur Quinney. "The Effects of Changes in Musculoskeletal Fitness on Health." *Canadian Journal of Applied Physiology* 26, no. 2 (2001): 161-216. doi:10.1139/h01-012.

13) Mann, Steven, Christopher Beedie, and Alfonso Jimenez. "Differential Effects of Aerobic Exercise, Resistance Training and Combined Exercise Modalities on Cholesterol and the Lipid Profile: Review, Synthesis and Recommendations." *Sports Medicine* 44, no. 2 (2013): 211-21. doi:10.1007/s40279-013-0110-5.

14) Hoff, Jan, Jan Helgerud, and Ulrik Wisløff. "Maximal Strength Training Improves Work Economy in Trained Female Cross-country Skiers." *Medicine & Science in Sports & Exercise* 31, no. 6 (1999): 870-77. doi:10.1097/00005768-199906000-00016.

15) Støren, Øyvind, Jan Helgerud, Eva Maria Støa, and Jan Hoff. "Maximal Strength Training Improves Running Economy in Distance Runners." *Medicine & Science in Sports & Exercise* 40, no. 6 (2008): 1087-092. doi:10.1249/mss.0b013e318168da2f.

16) Beattie, Kris, Brian P. Carson, Mark Lyons, Antonia Rossiter, and Ian C. Kenny. "The Effect of Strength Training on Performance Indicators in Distance Runners." *Journal of Strength and Conditioning Research* 31, no. 1 (2017): 9-23. doi:10.1519/jsc.0000000000001464.

17) Sato, Kimitake, and Monique Mokha. "Does Core Strength Training Influence Running Kinetics, Lower-Extremity Stability, and 5000-m Performance in Runners?" *Journal of Strength and Conditioning Research* 23, no. 1 (2009): 133-40. doi:10.1519/jsc.0b013e31818eb0c5.

18) Bliven, Kellie C. Huxel, and Barton E. Anderson. "Core Stability Training for Injury Prevention." *Sports Health: A Multidisciplinary Approach* 5, no. 6 (2013): 514-22. doi:10.1177/1941738113481200.

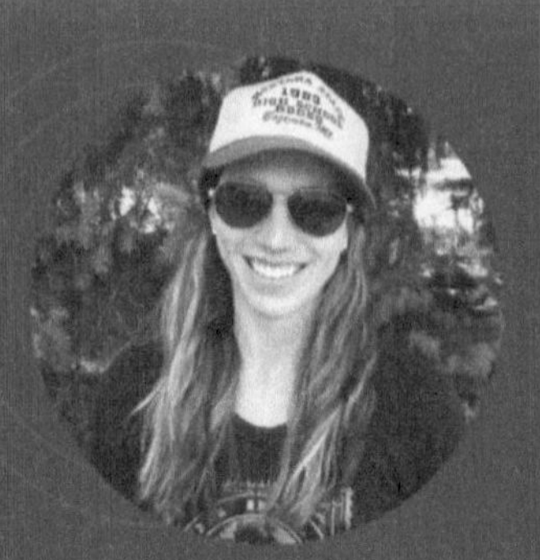

About Jen

INTERNATIONALLY UNKNOWN
AUTHOR JEN WEIR IS ON A
MISSION TO TAKE THE MYSTERY
OUT OF LIVING A HEALTHY LIFE.
AS AN EXPERIENCED CERTIFIED
STRENGTH & CONDITIONING
SPECIALIST, HEALTH COACH AND
PERSONAL TRAINER, JEN STRIPS
AWAY THE TWADDLE OF THE
HEALTH AND FITNESS INDUSTRY
TO HELP GIVE HER CLIENTS WHAT
THEY REALLY WANT — A NO-BS
APPROACH TO LIVING THE LIFE
THEY WANT. MOST OF THE TIME,
JEN HAS NO IDEA WHAT DAY IT IS,
IS IN DESPERATE NEED OF A
BEER AND A NAP, IS UP TO HER
NECK IN POOP (SHE RESIDES WITH
1 HUSBAND, 3 KIDS & 2 DOGS),
AND IS WORKING TENACIOUSLY TO
GET PEOPLE TO EAT REAL FOOD &
MOVE MORE.

www.ingramcontent.com/pod-product-compliance
Lightning Source LLC
Chambersburg PA
CBHW031919270726
48655CB00006BA/2824